Sonia's Feeling Sad

Sheila Hollins and Roger Banks
illustrated by Lisa Kopper

Books Beyond Words/RCPsych Publications
LONDON

13

15

22

The following words are for people who want a ready-made story rather than tell their own

1. Sonia's sister and husband come to visit with their new baby. Mum is excited to see them.

2. Mum clucks over the baby. Sonia feels left out.

3. Sonia runs out of the room. She is upset.

4. Sonia goes to bed and pulls the bedclothes around her. She is crying.

5. Mum wakes Sonia up. She says it's time to get up.

6. Sonia waits at the bus stop. She looks sad.

7. She's at her art class. Some people paint flowers, but Sonia paints everything black. Maybe this is how she feels.

8. After the class her friends go to a café. Sonia doesn't want to go.

9. Dinner at home and Sonia picks at her food.

10. It's the middle of the night. Sonia is in bed, and still awake. She can't sleep.

11. Sonia worries and tosses and turns. She still can't get to sleep.

12. In the morning mum tries to get her up. Sonia doesn't want to get up. She feels dreadful.

13. Mum takes her to the doctor. Mum and the doctor do all the talking. No one talks to Sonia.

14. The doctor takes blood from Sonia for a test. He wants to know what's wrong.

15. He gives a prescription to mum. Sonia doesn't understand what's happening.

16. Sonia is ready for bed. It's time to take the medicine. Sonia doesn't want to take it.

17. Sonia refuses to get up in the morning.

18. Mum takes her back to the GP.

19. This time the GP talks to Sonia. First he asks mum to wait outside.

20. He uses pictures of smiley and sad faces to find out how Sonia feels. She points at the sad picture. The GP listens to her and gives her some tissues to wipe her eyes.

21. The GP shows her this book to talk some more about how she feels.

22a. Sonia and mum go to meet a counsellor.

22. Sonia arrives at the counsellor's room with mum.

23. Sonia is on her own with the counsellor. The counsellor is listening.

24a. Sonia and her mum arrive at the clinic.

24. The counsellor says, 'Tell me more'.

25a. Mum and Sonia arrive for another appointment.

25. Sonia sees the counsellor again.

26a. Now Sonia comes to the clinic on her own.

26. Sonia draws a picture of her sister and her nephew. She looks happier.

27a. Sonia, mum and dad arrive at the clinic together.

27. The counsellor helps Sonia talk to her parents. Sonia tells them how she feels. They listen to her.

28. Sonia visits her sister and baby at home.

29. They take the baby for a walk together. Sonia pushes the buggy. What fun!

30. They stop for a drink and a chat. The baby is asleep now.

31. Sonia is at her art class again. She enjoys painting.

32. It's time for a picnic. Everyone smiles at Sonia. She is really better now. She doesn't feel sad any more.

33. Sonia feels great.

Introduction

This book is about a young woman with learning disabilities who becomes very sad and needs help to feel better.

Sadness and depression

Everyone can feel sad at any time in their lives, this is normal. There are things that happen, that people say or do, things that we think about that can make us all feel unhappy for a time. There are lots of words that people use for feeling this way: sad, unhappy, miserable, feeling blue, feeling down or low.

Although it is normal to feel this way, sometimes people may feel sad for longer than is usual and there may be other problems that come with this low mood.

When people are sad they find it difficult to see anything positive about their lives or their future. They may lose interest in doing things or may just not have the energy. They may cry a lot but they can also feel worried, unable to relax and irritable and impatient with others. For much of the time they may just feel empty, worthless or guilty. They can lose their appetite and have difficulty sleeping properly; though some people sleep or eat more than usual. Sometimes people may have physical symptoms such as stomach aches, bowel problems, headaches or other pains in the body and these can be related to the sadness they are feeling. Feelings of anxiety or panic are also common in people who are feeling sad.

If this sadness goes on for a long time, is quite severe and causes other problems – it becomes like an illness and doctors, psychiatrists and psychologists refer to this as 'depression'.

Some people are more likely to become depressed. It may come out of the blue or they may be someone who has a tendency to develop episodes of this low mood time after time. Sometimes you might be able to identify something that sets off this feeling.

In severe depression, a person can feel that life is meaningless and not worth living and have thoughts of wanting to harm themself or end their life.

Feelings are difficult things to describe and someone with learning disabilities or communication problems may not be able to tell other people how they feel and what they are thinking. Depression, therefore, shows in different ways such as changes in behaviour, losing the ability to do things or communicate with others, problems with control of bladder or bowel motions, angry outbursts, destructiveness or self-injury, and physical symptoms such as aches and pains.

Why do people with learning disabilities get sad or depressed?

People with learning disabilities will become sad and depressed for the same reasons as anybody else. There are some causes, however, that they might be more likely to encounter.

Loss and bereavement are commonly a cause for sadness and depression but not just when a family member or a friend dies. People who are supported by carers often have to cope with carers leaving; they may have been moved from one place to another in their lives, each time losing friends, carers, favourite and familiar activities and places. For an adult with learning disabilities who has lived with their parents all their life, when their parents die they not only have to face the loss of loved ones but they also may be moved into care and away from their home, familiar possessions and routines.

People with learning disabilities, as they grow up, can become very aware of how they are viewed and treated differently to people without learning disability. They see other young people having opportunities, responsibilities and achievements in life that they themselves have not been able or allowed to have and this can lead to feelings of disappointment, anger and sadness.

Sometimes physical health problems may be underlying a person's low mood, such as an underactive thyroid gland, viral infections, heart problems, pain in the joints, diabetes. We know, however, that people with learning disabilities are less likely to have their physical illnesses recognised and to be given treatment.

Neglect or physical and sexual abuse may lead to depression and people with learning disabilities are particularly at risk due to their dependency on others, difficulties in protecting themselves and not being able to speak up for themselves if abuse has happened.

Depression in women

After the age of 15, women are twice as likely as men to suffer from depression. There are lots of reasons why this happens. Girls and women may find that they are not given as much choice or opportunities in life by comparison with boys and men. They may be under pressure to take on roles in the family that are limiting and do not allow them to develop a sense of independence and freedom. Often, girls may end up having to care for a sick or disabled parent, to take on a lot of household tasks and their social and school life may suffer as a result. Like the young woman in this story, women with learning disabilities can find adolescence and early adulthood a difficult time when they see other people starting relationships, getting married and having children; they may feel that these are opportunities that they will not be able, or allowed, to have themselves.

It is also known that girls and young women, in particular those with learning disabilities, are more likely to be victims of sexual abuse and this can lead to great unhappiness and depression.

What to do if someone is sad or depressed

The most helpful thing to do is to help the person to talk about how they are feeling, to talk about what is on their mind and what things are troubling them. Often people will avoid talking to each other about unhappy or difficult feelings or particular problems or worries.

Being helped to talk these things through with a friend, supporter or member of the family can help to make sense of these difficulties and can also lead to finding some practical solutions to problems that have been underlying the sadness and worry.

Giving people information about sadness and depression and how to overcome them can be a great help. There are many books and websites that deal with these issues and some are in a form that is easier to read. This book without words is an example of something that can be given to a person to look at and to talk about with a friend or carer or in a group with other people who may have similar problems.

If the sad feelings continue then it is advisable for the person to see their general practitioner (GP). The doctor will check for any possible health problems that could be contributing to the depression, will investigate and treat these and also assist in finding other types of help if needed.

Because GPs usually only have short appointment times it is a good idea to explain when making a booking that more time may be needed. This is particularly important if the person with learning disabilities has communication problems and also if they are very nervous about seeing doctors. Extra time will help them to explain what has been happening and talk about things that it can be difficult to find the right words for.

It is always helpful for the person to be accompanied by someone who knows them well, who knows what sort of a person they usually are and who is able to explain how things have changed. It can also help to use pictures or drawings in trying to understand how someone has been feeling.

We must also remember that sometimes having someone else present can make it more difficult for the person to talk to the doctor. This may be the case when the person with learning disabilities wants to say things that might upset others, or if there is something that they want to keep private; people should always be allowed the opportunity to discuss their problems alone if they wish.

Help and treatment

For most types of depression, the GP will refer someone to see a counsellor or psychological therapist. The counsellor may see people at the doctor's surgery or they may have an office somewhere else. Counsellors offer people talking therapies, the opportunity to see them a number of times to talk about their feelings and problems that they have been having.

The counselling allows the person to talk about anything that they wish, including what has happened in their past. It will also focus on what thoughts they are currently having and how these might be making them feel worried or sad. For people with learning disabilities it is possible to adapt the therapy process to match the person's understanding or to help overcome problems in communication. Again, photographs or drawings or books like this one are very useful in helping people to understand each other better.

The counsellor, and the person they are helping, may decide that it would be helpful to meet with the person's family or carers to explain how the person has been feeling or particular problems that they have been having.

Occasionally, people may benefit from having a much longer course of talking therapy to work on difficult problems.

Although talking therapies are helpful for many people, they do not always improve the person's depression enough. In these cases, and for people who are severely depressed, a doctor can prescribe treatment in the form of antidepressant tablets or medicines; they can also give treatments for anxiety. These do not work for everybody and, if they do, it can take a few weeks of taking the treatment regularly before you notice a difference.

All tablets and medicines can have side-effects and treatments for depression and anxiety are no different; common ones are things like an upset stomach, diarrhoea, dizziness, difficulty sleeping or headaches. The doctor and/or pharmacist should give information on what kind of side-effects to expect, how most of them are not serious and may go away, and what to do if the side-effects are bad or causing significant problems and making the person feel worse. It is possible that changing to a different sort of treatment might be better.

If these treatments work, then it is important that the person does not stop taking them as soon as they stop feeling sad. It is necessary to keep taking the treatment for between 6 months and a year to make sure that the depression does not come back again.

People who do not get better with treatments from their GP, or whose depression is so bad that they are at risk through not eating or drinking enough or having strong thoughts about wanting to end their lives, can be referred to see a specialist. These specialists are called psychiatrists, and some have particular training and skills in working with people with learning disabilities; they usually work in teams of health professionals including nurses and psychologists.

Some people have depression that comes back time and again. If this is the case they will usually be seen by a psychiatrist, who, with the other members of the team, will provide a combination of both talking therapies and medicines that try to stop these episodes of depression from happening again, or make them more manageable.

Although sadness and depression are not a nice thing to have to go through, with the help of others this can often be a time for thinking about ways in which people want to change things in their lives. They can also deal with problems that have been around for a long time and think carefully about the changes they need to make that will help them to feel generally better about themselves and their life in the future.

Useful resources in the UK

(The information listed here was correct at time of publication.)

Organisations to contact for help and advice

Mencap's 'Getting it right' campaign (www.mencap. org.uk/gettingitright) helps people with learning disabilities get equal access to treatment. Mencap has worked with healthcare professionals and UK medical Royal Colleges to develop the 'Getting it right' charter, which lists the nine key adjustments that should be made for equal access to healthcare.

Mencap Learning Disability Helpline
If you have a problem accessing healthcare, you can contact this helpline on: 0808 808 1111

Typetalk: 18001 0808 808 1111
Text: 07717 989 029
Email: help@mencap.org.uk

MIND InfoLine: 08457 660 163 (local rate)
Available 9.15am to 5.15pm, Monday to Friday, for advice and support to service users.

Respond Helpline: 0800 808 0700
Supports people with learning disabilities, their carers and professionals, around any issue of trauma, including bereavement.

Samaritans: 08457 90 90 90 (local rate)
24-hour helpline for those feeling distressed,despairing or suicidal, or concerned about someone.
Email: jo@samaritans.org
Website: www.samaritans.org

Services in the UK

IAPT (Improving Access to Psychological Therapies)

In 2007 the English government made counselling available in primary care. IAPT was set up to find ways to improve the availability of psychological therapies, especially for people with depression or anxiety disorders. A document explaining how to access IAPT counsellors for people with learning disabilities is available at this website address: www.iapt.nhs.uk/wp-content/uploads/2009/02/83078-nhs-iapt-learning-dis.pdf

Community teams for people with learning disabilities (CTPLDs)

These are specialist multidisciplinary health teams that support adults with learning disabilities and their families by assessment, by supporting access to mainstream healthcare and by providing a range of clinical interventions, including counselling. Your GP or Social Services department should have the address of the local team.

Patient Advice and Liaison Service (PALS)

This service, known as PALS, has been introduced to ensure that the NHS listens to patients, their relatives, carers and friends, and answers their questions and resolves their concerns as quickly as possible. PALS also helps the NHS to improve services by listening to what matters to patients and making changes, when appropriate. Every hospital has a PALS service. You can contact them at your local hospital or via their website: www.pals.nhs.uk

Internet resources

Understanding Intellectual Disability and Health (www.intellectualdisability.info)

This website covers a wide range of physical and mental health issues for people with learning disabilities. It is designed for healthcare professionals and students but is widely used by family cares and support staff.

The Candle Project

The project offers guidance and resources to staff working with children and young people with learning disabilities and mental health issues. It makes links between a person's development and their culture, lifestyle, environment and mental health. A project resource is available free online (www.clearthoughts. info/silo/files/294.pdf) or you can purchase it as a book or CD from the Association for Real Change (www. arcuk.org.uk, email: david.grundy@arcuk.org.uk).

Depression in Adults with Intellectual Disability – Checklist for Carers (www.cddh.monash.org/ research/depression)

This Australian website allows free access to a checklist designed for use by carers, in particular paid support staff. It is intended to be used on behalf of adults who are not able to convey their feelings and symptoms because of severe communication impairment. It is not a diagnostic tool but the information can help the GP when considering the possibility that depression may be present. Details of how the Checklist can be used are also on the website.

What about us? (www.whataboutus.org.uk) supported some people with learning disabilities in mainstream schools to run action research projects about emotional well-being. They created an online resource which shares what they learned about how to support young people with learning disabilities.

Easy Health (www.easyhealth.org.uk) is a website created by Generate with easy to understand information about staying healthy and getting help with your health.

The following online resources are not specifically geared towards people with learning disabilities but might be useful to those with good literacy or their carers

Living Life to the Full (www.livinglifetothefull.com) is an online course offering a range of free educational life skills resources based on cognitive–behavioural therapy (CBT) principles.

MoodGYM (www.moodgym.anu.edu.au) is an Australian website which offers free self-guided resources for overcoming depression, including learning modules, assessments, an interactive game and downloadable relaxation audio materials.

The Australian website **depressioNet (www. depressionet.org.au)**, created by people with personal experiences of depression, aims to empower people to make informed choices and find solutions to the challenges of living with depression.

Beyond Blue (www.beyondblue.org.au) and **Youth Beyond Blue (www.youthbeyondblue.com)** are designed to help adults and young people with problems such as depression and anxiety.

Young Minds (www.youngminds.org.uk) work to improve the mental health of children and young people.

Written information

Mind booklets *Understanding Depression* and *Understanding Anxiety* can be purchased from www.mind.org.uk/shop/booklets

The **Mental Health Foundation** booklet *Dealing with Depression* (2006) helps people to recognise symptoms of depression and suggests remedies, including diet, exercise, medication and counselling. It can be downloaded for free from www.mhf.org.uk/publications.

An **Anxiety UK** booklet *The Carer's Guide to Anxiety* can be purchased at the Anxiety UK online shop: www.anxietyuk.org.uk/products/booklet/carers-guide-to-anxiety

A **Foundation for People with Learning Disabilities** booklet *All About Feeling Down* can be downloaded free from their website (www.learningdisabilities.org.uk/publications) or call Customer Services on 020 7803 1101.

CHANGE (www.changepeople.co.uk) has an illustrated booklet on depression for people with learning disabilities – *Depression. What is Depression? What Causes Depression? What Treatments are Available?*

You can order it from Change, Unit 41, Shine, Harehills Road, Leeds LS8 5HS. Telephone: 0113 388 0011.

Anxiety Disorders: The Caregivers – Information for Support People, Family and Friends by Kenneth Strong. ISBN 1590790561. Available from www.amazon.co.uk

Exploring Your Emotions Manual by A. Holland, A. Payne and L. Vickery. A set of 30 full-colour photographs illustrating common emotions that can be used in educational and therapeutic settings to help people with learning disabilities learn about their own feelings and the relationship between emotion and behaviour. Available from www.amazon.co.uk

Related titles in the Books Beyond Words series

Ron's Feeling Blue (2011) by Sheila Hollins, Roger Banks and Jenny Curran, illustrated by Beth Webb. This story is about a man who is depressed and shows how he is helped to feel better. New edition.

When Mum Died and *When Dad Died* (2004) are two books by Sheila Hollins and Lester Sireling, illustrated by Beth Webb. Both books take an honest and straightforward approach to death and grief in the family. The pictures tell the story of the death of a parent in a simple but moving way.

When Somebody Dies (2003) by Sheila Hollins, Noelle Blackman and Sandra Dowling, illustrated by Catherine Brighton. This book tells the story of two people who experience bereavements and the different support they are given.

Going to the Doctor (1996) by Sheila Hollins, Jane Bernal and Matthew Gregory, illustrated by Beth Webb. This book illustrates a variety of experiences which may occur during a visit to the GP. These include meeting the doctor, having one's ears syringed, a physical examination, a blood test, a blood pressure check and getting a prescription.

Some other titles in the Books Beyond Words series

Am I Going to Die? (2009) by Sheila Hollins and Irene Tuffrey-Wijne, illustrated by Lisa Kopper. This is a story about a man who is terminally ill, told in an honest and moving way.

I Can Get Through It (1998) by Sheila Hollins, Christiana Horrocks and Valerie Sinason, illustrated by Lisa Kopper. This story shows how a woman is helped to get through the experience of being abused with the help of a counsellor or therapist.

Jenny Speaks Out (2005) by Sheila Hollins and Valerie Sinason, illustrated by Beth Webb. Jenny feels unsettled when she moves into a new home in the community. Her carer and friends sensitively help Jenny to unravel her painful past as a victim of sexual abuse, to begin a slow but positive healing process.

Getting on with Cancer (2002) by Veronica Donaghy, Jane Bernal, Irene Tuffrey-Wijne and Sheila Hollins, illustrated by Beth Webb. This book tells the story of Veronica who has various treatments for cancer, including radiotherapy, chemotherapy and surgery. It deals honestly with the unpleasant side of treatment and ends on a positive note.

George Gets Smart (2003) by Sheila Hollins, Margaret Flynn and Philippa Russell, illustrated by Catherine Brighton. George's life changes when he goes running with his friends and workmates and he learns the importance of keeping clean and smart.

Michelle Finds a Voice (1997) by Sheila Hollins and Sarah Barnett, illustrated by Denise Redmond. Michelle has cerebral palsy and cannot communicate what she is feeling to the people who might help her. Michelle and her carers explore various solutions to overcome these difficulties, including the use of signing, symbol charts and electronic communication.

Falling in Love (1999) by Sheila Hollins, Wendy Perez and Adam Abdelnoor, illustrated by Beth Webb. This love story follows the relationship between Mike and Janet from their first date through to deciding to become engaged to be married.

Go to www.rcpsych.ac.uk/bbw for full details of all the titles available in the Books Beyond Words series.

You can purchase the books online or by writing to: Book Sales, Royal College of Psychiatrists, 17 Belgrave Square, London SW1X 8PG. Tel: 020 7235 2351 ext: 6146. Fax: 020 7245 1231.

Acknowledgements

We thank our editorial advisors Gary Butler, Sharon Jury, Kate Powell, Nigel Hollins, Robert Hill and Marion MacFarlane for their ideas and advice about what was needed in the pictures and to Jo Poynter from the Valuing People support team who arranged for the pictures to be trialled by individuals and groups.

We are grateful for the advice and support of our advisory group, which included representatives from Mind, the Judith Trust, Generate, the Challenging Behaviour Foundation and the Foundation for People with Learning Disabilities: Maria Jacovides, Joanna Brunt, Pam Vallance, Jane Pettingell, Vivien Cooper, Jill Davies, Julie Nixon, Annie Norman, Barbara Powell, Julia Garrett, Sonya Foley and Sandy Sherif. We thank all of the above for the time they gave most generously, including trialling the pictures with individuals and groups, and the experience they shared with us.

Thanks to Dorothea Duncan, who oversaw the project and gave of her time so generously, and Emily Westlake, who helped with the development of the book.

Finally, we are very grateful to the Department of Health for providing financial support for this book.

Authors

Sheila Hollins is Professor of Psychiatry of Learning Disability at St George's, University of London, and sits in the House of Lords. She is a past President and an Honorary Fellow of the Royal College of Psychiatrists.

Roger Banks is a Consultant in the Psychiatry of Learning Disability with Betsi Cadwaladr University Health Board. He is a Fellow of the Royal College of Psychiatrists and an Honorary Fellow of the Royal College of General Practitioners.

Lisa Kopper is a distinguished artist and illustrator of children's books. She is well known for her clear style and ability to draw feelings as well as form.